SPEED UP METABOLISM
How to lose weight in a short time

William Brandson

INTRODUCTION

Expanding the speed of your metabolism is most likely one of the least demanding and most ideal approaches to lose fat normally. Shape numerous individuals this may sound simple yet the best way to truly do this effectively is to roll out some way of life improvements that include eating routine and action levels. In a general public searching for the convenient solution this tends to fail to attract anyone's attention.

Metabolism is the procedure by which the body consumes calories to fuel its day by day works and is the procedure by which supplements in the nourishment we eat are separated in our cells to create vitality for these capacities. Metabolism is controlled by the thyroid organ in the neck, which thusly is administered by a piece of the mind called the hypothalamus. It is for the most part estimated by your basal metabolic rate (BMR), which is your resting metabolism.

Speeding up the metabolism makes a few advantages that will keep up weight loss advance. You will clearly accelerate the procedure at which your body changes over sustenance and put away fat into vitality and therefore you 'free weight'. You have to begin with your eating designs. Indeed, even a slight increment in your metabolic rate will accelerate fat loss over numerous months without strict abstaining from excessive food intake. By eating the best possible sustenance's and keeping up a decent exercise program you ought to have the capacity to accelerate your fat-consuming heater.

There are things you can do to rev up your metabolism, say nourishment specialists; similarly, as there are things that won't work by any stretch of the imagination. The possibility that fasting or skipping suppers regularly is an incredible method to wash down the arrangement of polluting influences, speed metabolism, and energize weight loss is simply one more legend. It might sound basic and exhausting, however justifiable reason adjusted eating regimens are what the nourishment specialists dependably suggest.

A standout amongst other approaches to speed your metabolism is with regular exercise joined with an eating routine suggested by sustenance specialists. Regular sustenance's with high nourishing quality take additionally preparing power (calories) to separate every one of those crucial supplements the body needs to keep running at top proficiency. Regardless you should have your general wellness and nourishment design in accordance with the objectives you need to accomplish and the more you think about how your body reacts to your way of life decisions, the better you can tweak a sustenance and exercise arrange for that is appropriate for you.

Doing the choice to get more fit is an intense activity, particularly in the event that you don't currently how to do it. By consolidating a solid and sensible eating routine alongside an exercise program you can start to speed your metabolism and begin getting more fit for all time.

Ways to Increase Metabolism With Foods That Speed Up Metabolism

Have you been hunting down approaches to build metabolism? or then again foods that speed metabolism? This will conceivably shock you. All foods speed metabolism.

"How could that be doable?" you inquire.

Give us a chance to take a quick look at just precisely what is metabolism, how it works, and the approaches to build metabolism. The accompanying conclusion may push you to much better comprehend the real procedure, and exactly how it might influence your framework.

At whatever point you eat a feast, your body initiates the procedure including processing the food, drawing out the genuine supplements and preparing every one of them to make vitality which keeps your body working legitimately and effectively.

It takes around 4 hours just to take in the supplements. This is rehashed with each feast you expend. In a day, that adds up to 12 hours that the body is dynamic retaining every feast's supplements.

Basically, amid the absorption procedure, our bodies consume calories. This is particularly valid for foods containing starches and protein, which as a rule take additional time than different foods to process. By utilizing these straightforward approaches to build metabolism of eating, processing and engrossing supplements from the food, you accelerate metabolism.

Does this suggest you have to eat significantly more to always empower calorie consuming?

Here's another answer on approaches to expand metabolism, that may astonish you. Indeed. In any case, hang on before you stop yourself before the cooler, kiddie apron set up, blade and fork primed and ready.

On the off chance that you skip breakfast and different suppers, you will moderate metabolism, or how rapidly your body consumes calories. We need to raise metabolism, and for this situation, devouring more food will help speed metabolism.

Quite eating downsized suppers all the more regularly amid the day, you can keep your metabolism working with the goal that your framework is always in the condition of calorie consumption.

As said, there are a few foods that require a greater amount of your body's vitality to consume. The genuine degree to which they affect your body's metabolism is reliant upon the specific food determination.

Foods That Speed Up Metabolism:

Caffeine, espresso, tea, chocolate and a compound substance found in chilies, are a few fixings that speed metabolism, however just negligible.

Metabolism promoters like carbs and protein trigger the most astounding rate of metabolism. All things considered a protein feast can consume as much as 25% of that dinner's calories by methods for assimilation and retention.

Despite the fact that a high protein supper may sound satisfying, consider that it would not offer your body with its required round of supplements. Counting vitamin and mineral supplements as approaches to build metabolism isn't the arrangement either, essentially in light of the fact that they don't give a similar nature of supplements that are discovered normally in foods.

The best decision is to devour very much adjusted foods that accelerate metabolism on a regular premise which contain protein, non-dull vegetables, fats and starches. This will reduce fat creation while protecting your glucose at a degree that consumes fat and construct muscle.

Focus on these Top 10 particular foods that successfully accelerate metabolism and consume off fat.

Top Ten:

- Entire grain bread

- Chicken

- Salmon

- Eggs

- New Cheese

- Green Beans

- Summer Squash

- Cabbage

- Asparagus and other non-bland vegetables.

Also, obviously, protein rich meats.

To briefly help your metabolic rate by as much as 30%, drink icy water.

Keep in mind, there are different components outside your ability to control that will affect your body's speed of metabolism, including your age, sex, and any therapeutic conditions.

While these kinds of foods can speed metabolism, the most ideal approach to get more fit is with a solid blend of regular dinners and exercise, particularly those that construct muscle just in light of the fact that muscle consumes calories as well.

Exercise on a regular premise, stay with an eating regimen of protein, non-dull vegetables, fats and starches, and make certain you include a portion of those foods that speed metabolism, and you'll soon observe the impacts you need.

Are you flabby, somewhat heavier than you might want to be, or maybe wellness has moved toward becoming too tedious, and has transformed into something more like work to you.

At that point you will need to look at this wellness elective, that is helpful, financially savvy, eliminates time imperatives, and all from the solace of your own home.

Customizing Your Own Nutritional Plan Through the Metabolic Typing Diet

As indicated by the defenders of the metabolic composing diet, every individual has his own one of a kind healthful necessities. Obviously, our disparities in metabolism call for changing dietary needs. Distinguishing the metabolic sort will enable you to comprehend why keeping up a low-starch diet might be advantageous for a few people while the same nutritious esteem might be undesirable for others.

To start with presented by William Kelly in 1960, metabolic composing is centered around one's dietary decisions in light of the exercises of the sensory system. While he kept on advancing such dietary framework, Harold Kristal and William Wolcott additionally built up the training. It turned into the reason for the change of nutritious sort.

Metabolic writing is a mind-boggling procedure of distinguishing the fitting mix of supplements which is viewed as extraordinary to each person. Keep in mind that each individual varies with regards to wholesome prerequisites. All together for the body to work well, there must be an adequate supply of supplements which incorporate protein, fat, minerals, vitamins, starches and water. These fundamental substances will guarantee that every single substantial capacity are completed appropriately.

Presently if the cells in our body don't get the correct supplements, they won't have the capacity to play out their capacity well. Therefore, inability to perform different substance responses in the body may result to incessant infections, for example, liver issue, diabetes and malignancy. As per contemplates, off-base mix of supplements does not enable the cells to work suitably. In spite of the fact that you might get a few starches and protein, off-base blend of these substances will most likely be unable to fuel the cells.

Lacking and mistaken mix of supplements may not just affect one's wellbeing at a cell level. On the off chance that you know precisely your metabolic sort, you will have the capacity to legitimately bolster the nutritious needs of your body. You may most likely end up making the inquiry, "What is the best diet for me"? Indeed, it just takes one thing to have the capacity to your body with the correct blend of supplements and that is by distinguishing your metabolic or healthful compose.

What is Your Metabolic Type?

Through the metabolic writing diet, you will have the capacity to effortlessly distinguish the most reasonable diet for your body. William Wolcott ordered contrasts in metabolism into three gatherings.

a. Protein Type. This metabolic sort is viewed as quick oxidizers. In the event that you are a protein write, you may ache for salty and greasy foods. Visit yearning may likewise be experienced as your body may consume more starches too rapidly. High-fat protein diet works best for individuals under this metabolic kind.

b. Carbo Type. In spite of the main metabolic write, carbo types have a tendency to have poor hungers. Keeping in mind the end goal to accelerate the oxidation rate, expanded sugar admission might be required. Carbo writes are exceedingly prescribed to keep up a low-protein diet. Their day by day healthful arrangement ought to incorporate direct measure of sugars and low-fat dairy products.

c. Blended Type. In the event that an individual is a blended kind, he is likely in the middle of the two metabolic classes. Since there is a metabolic unevenness which is the reason there is a requirement for a direct blend of protein and sugar-rich foods.

Raising Your Metabolism - Secret To The Metabolism

The procedure of metabolism is critical and changes over food into vitality or fuel. At that point the body utilizes these for everyday exercises. It additionally includes the procedure of capacity of fat, which is later changed over to energy. So what is the key to the metabolism and raising your metabolism? There are essentially two sorts of individuals. One is individuals who have a quick metabolism. These individuals have no issue in consuming calories and store less fat. Then again there are individuals who have a moderate metabolism. These individuals have an issue consuming calories and store more fat that is important. For individuals who have a moderate metabolism, raising your metabolism is vital for weight loss. There are some who have been determined to have metabolic scatters and maturing becomes possibly the most important factor when we are raising your metabolism. Factors for Raising Your metabolism raising your metabolism accurately and successfully, you should comprehend the body's metabolic needs and what number of calories it employment. The metabolic needs are the measure of vitality required for the body to work every day.

Calories then again, are the measure of calories consumed amid these substantial capacities, for example, moving, running reasoning and more. Raising your metabolism or expanding your metabolism has a ton to do with your metabolic rate. How well does your body do at playing out your typical metabolic undertakings? While expanding metabolism, you have to decide your "resting or basal metabolic rate." This will change starting with one individual then onto the next. This metabolic rate is the measure of calories you consume that your body needs to keep tissues and organs working legitimately. A decent govern is the greater you are the more calories you have to play out these processes. Raising your metabolism isn't that simple. There are distinctive variables that decide a man's metabolic rate, so you need to utilize diverse ways to deal with increment your metabolism. Genes have an imperative part in this condition. A few people are conceived with quick metabolisms and other have a moderate metabolism. Age is another factor when attempting to make sense of how to accelerate metabolism.

As individuals get more established the measure of calories required decreases. Another factor to raising your metabolism is what are your physical movement and your muscle improvement. A successful path in raising your metabolism is exercise. This will elevate your body to use quicker. This speedier metabolism even happens after you have finished the exercise. Individuals who have great muscle advancement will build their metabolism quicker than individuals who don't'. The purpose behind this is more muscles consume more calories effectively. Nutrition is another incredible method for speeding up your metabolism. This includes the correct supply of various supplements, regular exercise and perhaps a way of life change. Raising your metabolism works this way. Lose some weight, you will need to treat metabolic clutters. Endeavor to stop the indications of maturing by keeping your metabolism at ordinary levels. For more data on Metabolism Disorders and the right method of raising your metabolism

An Overview of the New Metabolic Typing Diet

Not at all like most diets today, this diet is outlined in your body's exceptional dietary needs - a kind of altered arrangement. In case you're becoming weary of customary diets, you might be charmingly amazed at this one of a kind diet design. It might be only the thing you have to help your weight loss for good.

Allows first investigate customary diets. A large portion of them can be categorized as one of 3 classes - the low-fat diet, the high-protein diet, or the adjusted, calorie-inadequate diet. Wholesome specialists have differed for quite a while with respect to what diet is ideal, leaving a significant number of us more confounded than any other time in recent memory. More awful yet, unnerve strategies are regularly utilized, abandoning us dreading for our lives. Maybe it's chance that we found out about the newfound metabolic writing diet, as the other option to these plans.

So where's the science behind this metabolic writing? It started with dental practitioner Weston Price while voyaging broadly. He was considering individuals of changing societies and found the connection between present-day dietary patterns and endless degenerative ailments. He saw there was a particular connection between's the individuals who ate a diet similar to their precursors and the high level of wellbeing and wellness that resulted. In any case, he likewise saw an aggravating theme among populaces that moved. These gatherings were appeared to be not well prepared to process this new assortment of foods productively, and these populaces frequently hinted at diminished imperativeness. Today, with the amounts of prepared foods that we devour, pandemic extents of overweight, heftiness, and a large group of present-day sicknesses torment our general public. Hereditary and natural factors appear in our metabolism, and we think that its difficult to get in shape unless we re-adjust to help our hereditary needs.

How about we See How the Metabolic Typing Diets Work: The idea driving this arrangement is that every individual's metabolism capacities contrastingly with regards to these 2 factors:

1. Autonomic sensory system strength. At the end of the day, we monitor vitality and process food in the parasympathetic sensory system, though we consume vitality in the thoughtful sensory system - where the "battle or flight" hormones lives. Researchers who examine this sort of diet trust that

every individual inclines more toward one end of the vitality consuming range.

2. The rate at which you consume calories. A few of us are moderate oxidizers, who change over food into vitality at a slower rate. Keeping in mind the end goal to adjust their frameworks, they do best on the off chance that they center around carbohydrates instead of protein and fat. Other individuals are quick oxidizers who change over food into vitality rapidly. With a specific end goal to adjust their frameworks, quick oxidizers need to eat heavier proteins and fats to enable them to balance out how rapidly they consume their vitality.

On the off chance that you need to take in your metabolic sort, there are a couple of choices accessible. For outright precision, a prepared wellbeing expert can give an entire evaluation, which regularly incorporates pee and blood tests. For a large portion of us, in any case, a straightforward individual test that you take at home can frequently distinguish your metabolic kind. One such test solicits you an arrangement from 15-20 questions encompassing your eating inclinations and examples.

There are three general metabolic types:

Protein types - Protein types - ought to eat a diet that is richer in fats, protein, and oils, and in addition organ meats or other quality proteins, while carbohydrate ought to bring down are quick oxidizers. As such they consume fuel rapidly. They have a tendency to be as often as possible hungry, ache for greasy, salty foods, fizzle with low-calorie diets, and tend towards exhaustion, tension, and anxiety. They are frequently torpid or feel "wired", "nervous", with shallow vitality while being worn out underneath.

Carbo types - Carbo types - should center around foods that are high in carbohydrates and low in fats, proteins, and oils. They are moderate oxidizers, who consume fuel gradually. They, by and large, have generally feeble cravings, a high resistance for desserts, issues with weight administration, "type An" identities, and are frequently reliant on caffeine.

Blended types - Mixed types are someplace amidst the other two types. They, for the most part, have normal hunger, longings for desserts and boring foods, the generally little issue with weight control, and tend towards exhaustion, tension, and apprehension. Individuals with this write ought to eat a blend of high-fat, proteins, and eggs, cheese, yogurt, tofu, and nuts in break even with sums.

For some individuals, this remarkable diet has demonstrated to explain the riddle to their weight loss needs. If you are disappointed in light of the fact that nothing appears to work for you, it may be justified regardless of your while to look advance into the metabolic composing design.

The Difference Between Type I and Type II Diabetes Mellitus

The vast majority of the general population these days understand that there are two sorts of diabetes mellitus, in any case, what number of us really understand that the refinement between two of them? Following is a snappy review of the two types and precisely clarifies how they show themselves.

Type I diabetes can be known as insulin-subordinate diabetes mellitus and it is the impact of an absence of insulin emission inside the explore different avenues regarding cells of your pancreatic. It may be the way that tries different things with tissues have been decimated by the infection like a disease or even an immune system condition and along these lines, their own working can be altogether diminished. Now and again, in any case, there will presumably be an acquired propensity that prompts beta cell crumbling and furthermore look into demonstrates that a nearby individual from the family has around 1/20 shot of also creating type I diabetes while the likelihood inside the general population is around 1/250.

The most widely recognized beginning of type I diabetes is as a rule around 14 years of age and furthermore, almost all of the influenced people are normally clinically decided preceding their twentieth birthday celebration. It might create rapidly finished an era of half a month or possibly days and furthermore appears alone all through the adhering to 3 stage designs:

The first is expanded blood glucose. The second one has quickened usage of muscle versus fat with respect to power and for the creation in regards to cholesterol through the liver organ. The third one is decimation in the body's proteins dealers

This will display ostensibly by utilizing a sudden drop in whole body muscle estimate which isn't stopped in spite of in the case of ingesting a lot of foods. A patient will probably understand totally worn and normally sickly conditions.

Type I diabetes may be treated with the hormone insulin and that is infused using, and the hormone is insulin tube. Giving you where your situation is uncovered decently fast and the diabetic settings their diet program and furthermore insulin medications, at that point there is no justifiable reason motivation behind why they can continue going life as ordinary.

Type II diabetes is significantly more across the board than class I, representing 80-90% with respect to recognized occasions including diabetes. In numerous occurrences, the time of approaching is 40+ decades with almost all remaining clinically analyzed identifying with the age gatherings of 50 and 60. Instead of type I, this type creates little by pretty much nothing and can visit unnoticed for a long time.

Type II diabetes is too distinguished as non-insulin, depending diabetes mellitus (NIDDM) is an outcome from a decreased level of affectability with respect to objective structures to the metabolic connection between the hormone insulin. This sort of decreased level of affectability can frequently be alluded to as insulin level of opposition.

By and large type II diabetes might be basically treated, albeit still at the early levels, alongside a caloric administered diet design and furthermore delicate exercise to promote fat diminishment. Now and again, medications might be utilized that raise insulin affectability or maybe result in the pancreas to discharge additional degrees of blood insulin. In the event that your ailment advances, at that point blood insulin supervision is regularly required to direct blood glucose.

The two types of diabetes mellitus are genuinely genuine illnesses and should be managed in this way. Awful activities will cause a diabetic example in cases staying unchecked, diabetic individual unconsciousness and loss of life.

What's the Difference Between Type 1 Diabetes and Type 2 Diabetes?

Diabetes is a metabolic issue portrayed by high glucose and different indications. With this issue, the beta cells of the pancreas can't deliver enough insulin to control glucose levels. There are two principal types of diabetes, type 1 and type 2. Type 1 is caused by an immune system response in the pancreas. Type 2 is described by insulin opposition and can advance to the loss of beta cell work. The two types are serious incessant conditions, however, are treatable with insulin infusions and dietary changes.

Type 1 diabetes is caused by a loss of beta cells in the pancreas, which prompts an insulin inadequacy. What causes the beta cell loss is a T-cell intervened immune system assault. The chief treatment is supplanting insulin in the body. Without insulin, genuine manifestations, trance-like state, and even demise can come about. To date, there are no precaution techniques known for type 1. 10% of all diabetics in North American and Europe have this type of diabetes. This type was initially called "adolescent diabetes", because of a lion's share of cases being kids. Type 1 diabetes can be treated with insulin and checked by utilizing glucose meters. Diet and exercise can help in the administration of this issue. Treatment ought not to meddle with typical exercises, insofar as there is adequate mindfulness, proper care and train taken in testing and taking endorsed meds.

Type 2 diabetes comes about because of a blend of deficient insulin emission and insulin obstruction or decreased insulin affectability. In spite of the fact that the correct reason for type 2 is obscure, it appears that focal stoutness inclines individuals for insulin obstruction, potentially in view of hormone emissions that disable glucose resilience. Fifty-five percent of people with type 2 diabetes are large. Maturing and family history additionally appears to assume apart at the beginning of this type. Type 2 diabetes is first treated by diet and exercise, which can re-establish insulin affectability. A few diabetics can control their glucose levels just by these normal techniques. On the off chance that this doesn't work, the following stage is treated with oral insect diabetic medications. In the event that the oral meds fall flat, insulin treatment will be actualized.

What Are Metabolic Types?

The acknowledgment of various Metabolic Types started with the perceptions of a dental specialist, Weston Price, who voyaged everywhere throughout the world in the 1930s and was flabbergasted at the colossal contrasts in diet that he saw. Considerably all the more intriguing was the way that where a clan or individuals had been generally disengaged and had built up a quite certain diet, occurrences of most degenerative sicknesses and illnesses were relatively incredible. Drawn out great wellbeing was particularly the standard.

Anyway, he soon understood that it was not just an instance of managing that, "we should all eat like the Inuit for wellbeing and lifespan!" The high fat and protein diet of the tough and sound Inuit was in complete difference to the organic product, vegetable and grain-rich diets of the seemingly perpetual, sharp and dynamic Mediterranean villagers, or the rice and vegetable diet of the East Asians. Indeed, he perceived that there were numerous variables that separated the different clans and people groups.

Yet, one thing he recognized and which has been demonstrated over and over from that point onward, is that our advanced western diet runs as an inseparable unit with a wide range of medical issues and issues.

His perceptions fascinated different researchers, similar to George Watson, Roger Williams and William Kelly, who all kept on looking into this territory. They arrived at the conclusion that there are two primary factors that decide how our bodies respond to the food we eat, and that these are mostly controlled by our hereditary legacy:

1. Which autonomic sensory system is predominant - There are two branches to this framework, the thoughtful sensory system and the parasympathetic sensory system. The main gives us our "battle or flight" intuition, consumes vitality quickly and stifles the stomach related framework. The parasympathetic framework then again quiets us down, spare vitality and process food completely. The researchers reached the conclusion that whichever of these two frameworks was prevailing would impact how our bodies procedure the food we put into them.

2. The rate of cell oxidation - at the end of the day the speed with which our cells tend to transform food into vitality. On the off chance that we are quick oxidizers, at that point, our bodies change over food rapidly into vitality. It's prescribed that quick oxidizers eat a lot of overwhelming proteins and fats which take more time to separate and discharge vitality. Moderate oxidizers then again require a diet construct more with respect to carbohydrates which discharge their vitality all the more rapidly.

33

In spite of the fact that these are the two principle factors under thought, metabolic writing assumes that we are each a one of a kind blend of these and different elements, in an individual biochemical outline. William Walcott and Trish Fahey, in their book "The Metabolic Typing Diet" incorporate a straightforward test to decide comprehensively where we fit on the metabolic range. The result of the test places every one of us to differing degrees in one of three principle metabolic types:

The Protein Metabolic Type - every now and again ravenous, aches for salty, greasy foods and has issues overseeing vitality levels - either built up or lazy.

The Carbohydrate Metabolic Type- once in a while extremely ravenous and can go for quite a while on generally little food. Pines for desserts and sugary foods. Frequently has weight administration issues.

Blended Metabolic Type - as the name proposes, this metabolic type is someplace in the middle of the other two, with a few attributes from every one of alternate types. Frequently has low vitality and high uneasiness.

When you know which wide metabolic type you fit into, a by and large helpful diet can be arranged, however, for the best outcomes, an unmistakably nitty gritty investigation will decide precisely what blend of supplements and food types will make them work at ideal productivity.

14 Surprising Ways to Increase Your Metabolism to Lose Weight and Boost Energy

Metabolism is the procedure that separates the food we eat to deliver the vitality our bodies need to work. The body utilizes vitality for all that it does; eating, resting and notwithstanding breathing requires vitality. So we are continually consuming calories to make vitality.

In the event that your metabolism is moderate, it isn't working at ideal levels and less of your calories will get transformed into vitality. A few things that may make you have a moderate metabolism are; not getting enough exercise, age, hereditary qualities, and what and when you eat. Signs of a moderate metabolism can incorporate inclination frosty, dry skin, obstruction, low pulse, and exhaustion. Likewise, weight pick up and not having the capacity to get in shape could be indications of a moderate metabolism.

Our metabolism backs off as we get more seasoned. Some say it starts moderating as ahead of schedule at age 25. Expanding your metabolism implies consuming more calories which rise to more vitality. This has numerous medical advantages. Essentially it will profit all your body's capacities that require vitality, which is every one of them. It can give you more vitality amid the day and help you rest around evening time, it can likewise enable you to get to a solid weight, and remain there.

Exercise is an incredible method to build your metabolism and presumably the most widely recognized. Recorded beneath are some different ways that have been accounted for to build metabolism alongside more data on everyone.

Eat 5-7 times each day

As you eat and process food your body utilizes more vitality and in this manner consumes more calories. Eating regularly will likewise keep your glucose stable which will build your metabolism. Both skipping suppers and not getting enough calories back off your metabolism.

Fabricate muscle;

Muscle requires more vitality to keep up than fat does. So on the off chance that you increment your bulk, your metabolism will accelerate to create more vitality which implies consuming more calories.

Having breakfast;

Studies recommend that having breakfast can expand your resting metabolism by 10%. Having breakfast can support your vitality, lessen hunger, and advance better decisions for the duration of the day. Skipping breakfast backs off your metabolism.

Vitamin B;

B vitamins assume a noteworthy part in the metabolism of fat, proteins, and carbohydrates. The body needs B12 to deliver sound red platelets which are essential to vitality production. The body utilizes Vitamin B12 for the majority of its metabolic procedures. Vitamin B12 has been accounted for to be the main consideration in deciding your Basal Metabolic Rate. Basal Metabolic Rate is the measure of vitality you utilize while very still. B12 additionally benefits the mind and sensory system.

Vitamin C;

Scientists at the University of Colorado at Boulder announced that vitamin C may build metabolism by diminishing oxidative worry from responses in the body. Oxidative pressure is accepted to back off your metabolism and increments with age. Vitamin C likewise helps bolster the safe framework and can wreck unsafe microbes and infections.

Cinnamon;

Test thinks about done by the U.S. Horticulture Service found that a dynamic compound in cinnamon builds metabolism. Different investigations propose cinnamon can bring down LDL cholesterol and manage glucose.

Chromium;

Chromium controls the sugar metabolism in the body and is required for the metabolism of fats, proteins, and carbohydrates. Chromium Picolinate has been said to expand metabolism, and decrease food cravings, and sweet longings.

Chuckling;

Analysts at Vanderbilt University in Nashville, Tennessee, found that chuckling can expand your metabolism by 10 to 40 calories. Giggling can likewise bring down circulatory strain and lessen pressure hormones like cortisol and adrenaline.

Rest;

When we rest our bodies create larger amounts of development hormone which builds metabolism. Rest has likewise been accounted for to battle coronary illness, soothe pressure, help your memory, and lessen your hazard for sadness.

Daylight;

UVB wavelengths have been accounted for to fire up the metabolic and synthetic procedures that deliver vitamin D. Reports propose that daylight can build metabolism, mitigate wretchedness, and enhance assimilation.

Water;

An examination done in Germany demonstrated a 30% expansion in the resting metabolism rate of subjects who drank 500ml of water a day. It has been accounted for that our bodies require no less than some water to work appropriately at a fundamental level.

Ice;

Typical body temperature is around 98.6 degrees. Our bodies are continually attempting to remain at that temperature. When we eat or drink things that are cool, our metabolism increments to create the vitality to warm us move down.

Magnesium;

The atom that gives vitality to every metabolic procedure is found in magnesium. Magnesium is required for the metabolism of fats and carbohydrates. It has likewise been accounted for help direct circulatory strain and to help fortify bones, and teeth.

Metabolism composing;

It has been recommended that every individual has a particular metabolism, generally one of three types. This type figures out which foods advantage your metabolism and which ones don't. In this way, one sort of food could give one individual vitality and help them to shed pounds, yet make someone else tired and make them pick up or shield them from losing any weight, contingent upon their metabolism type. Discovering which type you are enables you to know which foods to eat a greater amount of, which ones to eat less of and which ones to maintain a strategic distance from on the off chance that you need to upgrade your metabolism to help your vitality, get in shape, and have the capacity to keep it off.

8 Signs You Should Invest In Your Health

With regards to examining about investing in your health, there are a couple of essential angles that ought to be mulled over. Following are 8 signs you ought to put resources into your health:

1. You are confronting trouble in nodding off or strolling up

Rest term can influence metabolic and neurological capacities that are basic to the upkeep of person's health. Rest issue are frequently connected with a higher danger of coronary illness, diabetes, pulse, and corpulence. Satisfactory rest is important to battle against contamination, do well at school or work, and enhance the digestion of sugar to overt diabetes. Because of absence of rest, day by day routine can endure, including comprehension, inclinations, and memory.

2. You are coming up short your tests

Terrible aftereffects of cholesterol, adrenal pressure, glucose, thyroid levels, and circulatory strain tests would all be able to point to the way that adjustments in your eating routine are required. Nourishment is the key prerequisite for healthy living. Furthermore, you should know how to execute those progressions.

3. You are having cerebral pains, or are frequently becoming ill

These days, thinking about the chaotic workplace, having a migraine, or back agony could undoubtedly go unnoticed as a sign of "working too hard," or even "routine issue". That is, in any case, a misnomer. Affliction and torment is a reasonable sign that something isn't right with your body. On the off chance that you overlook signs your body gives, they get conspicuous with more agony that is unending, including repeating diseases, headaches, and body torment. The principal thing you have to do is to recover your eating on track, since it is a standout amongst the most vital components of your health.

4. You are going out to eat regularly, or don't recognize what to plan for supper

These days, individuals have built up the inclination of consuming more sustenances arranged from home than any time in recent memory. They are of the view that it requires such a great amount of investment to cook. Be that as it may, always eating takeout nourishment implies spending stacks of cash and harming your health. It isn't that hard to cook at home. All you require is legitimate arranging. Once an arrangement is actualized, you will discover that it doesn't require much investment to cook.

5. You are stressed over your unreasonable body weight or body picture

Having great sustenance is basic to effective weight administration. According to an examination report, abstain from food controls around 75 percent of weight misfortune. Clearly, exercise and development is urgent to weight misfortune, yet sustenance is generally the primary factor.

On the off chance that you keep on eating low-calorie sustenances or take after prohibitive eating intends to decrease weight, it will just prompt poor outcomes, subsequently making hormonal awkward nature, moderate digestion, and so forth.

6. You are skipping suppers regular

On the off chance that you are frequently missing dinners, it is a sign you have to concentrate more on your health. Regardless of whether coincidentally or intentionally, skipping dinners isn't the most ideal approach to get more fit. Skipping dinners can prompt the improvement of diabetes, deficient nourishment, and other health difficulties. In the event that you are hoping to shed pounds, make a point not to skip suppers. So as to effectively shed pounds, it is essential to keep your digestion working with the correct nourishment. Skipping dinners makes individuals hungrier and they in the long run compensate for the lost calories in any case. You have to take in the best possible approach to fuel your body.

7. You don't know what is healthy

The way that there is a great deal of clashing data accessible out there makes it amazingly intense to make sense of what is healthy. In the event that you have confronted this quandary, at that point think about yourself in the larger part. The normal individual isn't sure about what makes up an ideal eating routine. One wellspring of this disarray can be credited to the huge measure of nourishment data that individuals are presented to.

8. Your face does not look new and scarcely discernible differences show up on your skin

When you begin seeing scarcely discernible differences on your skin, you should realize that something isn't right. These lines might be an indication of maturing skin, and can influence you to look more seasoned than what you really are. So as to manage this issue, ensure that your eating routine is brimming with vitamin A, C, and zinc.

All things considered, regardless of whether these signs are not showing up yet, you have to guarantee a healthy and adjusted eating routine. Avoidance is constantly superior to cure.

What Are the Effective Ways to Raise Your Metabolism?

Our bodies get the imperativeness we require from sustenance through absorption, which are the compound reactions in the body's cells that change over the fuel from support into the essentialness anticipated that would do everything from theory to moving from place to put. Kick start your day with two direct lifestyle affinities that will encourage your processing. Practicing toward the beginning of the day at an energetic pace for around 10 minutes, for instance - skipping, lively strolling or cycling tough for 10 minutes, which will put your digestion into high apparatus, and with "max engine propulsion" impact of a vivacious exercise keeps your digestion high for whatever is left of the day. Have a healthy breakfast with the blend of lean protein and fiber supper from "The Diet Solution" formulas which will keep you from eating all the more later in the day and unexpectedly get your digestion working by separating the sustenance that was devoured.

You should dependably go for 30 to 45 minutes of activity every day, 5 days seven days to keep your digestion in an abnormal state. One of these techniques is to practice in 10-minute interims at four to five times each day to build your digestion for the duration of the day. Our body muscles consume a larger number of calories than fat, weight preparing each other day assembles fit bulk and this is extraordinary compared to other approaches to build your digestion. When you add more muscle to your body, you are consuming more calories, bringing about snappier fat misfortune. A healthy eating regimen will help keep your vitality up so you can keep working out. Littler dinners around four to five times each day with bunches of leafy foods, alongside lean protein, nuts, and entire grains, will guarantee your digestion remains lifted.

Remaining dynamic and move additionally amid the day by taking part in the incremental exercise, for example, taking the stairs, stopping the auto assist away, and strolling someplace as opposed to driving will support your digestion. Get quality seven hours of rest every day, which is a critical time for the body to rest and reenergize.

Drink eight to ten glasses of water for each day, which keeps you hydrated, especially since you are accomplishing more exercise, and it likewise mimics a sentiment completion. Your digestion will moderate when you are got dried out.

By figuring out how to manage stress or attempt to evade stress inside and out by expelling yourself from stressful circumstances will keep up your body's vitality levels, endeavor to set aside a brief period every day or requiring significant investment off to make the most of your side interest or participating in most loved leisure activity, for example, cultivating or taking your puppy for a stroll to get away from the weights of life.

Five Shocking Revelations Exposing Why Metabolic Disorders Causes Acute Obesity!

Statement:

"While weight loss is essential, what's more, vital is the nature of sustenance you put in your body - nourishment is data that rapidly changes your digestion and qualities.

Today might be your day of reckoning. Why? You inquire! Since, this day I am here to get out the weight loss amusement put away, open it, unfurl the direction and lay it out for you, a sharp calorie counter like yourself. The lead on this diversion depends on metabolic disorder confound of how unfriendly sustenance responses influence our weight, by implication! Trust me, this stripped truth can't be overemphasized. With no shadow of uncertainty sustenance, hypersensitivities and sensitivities contribute emphatically to a few calamitous disorders of digestion: And digestion assume a vital part of weight loss!

Before we continue to the diagram of this chapter, let me accentuation that metabolic disorder is the lynchpin in the round of life of weight loss and so on.

Outline:

It resembles plunging your toes to get a vibe of the strange waters. That is the key issues that influence our weight loss endeavors. To put it plainly, the metabolic disorder causes:

• The hormonal irregularity of the endocrine framework.

• Disturb insulin levels,

• Cause mind-set science disturbances.

• Energy and safe brokenness.

• Candida (unsafe parasites) b yeast colonization in mucosal layers

Hi! Is it accurate to say that you are still with me up until this point? Try not to stress! Regardless of whether you're not, simply continue perusing. You will at last snatch the whole idea of this chapter, Believe me!

Right away, let start with the principal disorder! Should we?

Disorder No. 1. The hormonal lopsidedness of the endocrine framework.

Basically, they meddle with the hormonal adjust of the endocrine framework. This obviously incorporates the thyroid and adrenal organs. This makes it harder for the body to bum put away fat.

Next, how about we move along to disorder no 2 which is it bothers insulin levels. Then again do keep in your mind why again that hormonal unevenness of the endocrine framework can and will make it harder for the body to burn stored fats. Concur?

Disorder No. 2. They bother insulin levels!

Without question, explore have discovered that even in individuals who can keep up an ordinary capacity of the thyroid and adrenals. This flags the body to change over nourishment vitality into fat and furthermore adds to hypoglycemia.

The following disease is none other than, Disorder No. 3. They cause temperament science interruptions.

Trust it or not, sustenance responses really cause levels of the quieting neurotransmitter serotonin to fall, prompting despondency, uneasiness, and urgent eating urges, all of which generally trigger gorging. Serotonin shakiness additionally compounds numerous physical disorders, including headaches, menstrual disorder, fibromyalgia, and peevish gut disorder. These troublesome conditions regularly upset good dieting designs.

How about we give a boisterous yell to disorder number four. Okay?

Disorder No. 4. They cause vitality and safe brokenness.

Nourishment hypersensitivities and sensitivities extraordinarily diminish vitality, add to a sleeping disorder, and dis-direct resistance (since sustenance responses are generally glitches of the invulnerable reaction). Every one of the three of these issues meddles extraordinarily with the capacity, to work out. They likewise contribute notably to the beforehand said metabolic disorders.

At long last, Disorder No. 5. Candida yeast colonization in mucosal layers.

Notwithstanding all the above, nourishment hypersensitivities and sensitivities in a roundabout way add to the event of candida (unsafe growths) yeast colonization in mucosal films, which causes symptoms like those of ceaseless weariness disorder and causes swelling. Lamentably, yeast colonization at that point compounds unfriendly sustenance responses.

Metabolic Disorders and Diabetes

Metabolic disorders are generally hereditary conditions that influence the generation of vitality inside the cells; in any case, some happen because of ill-advised eating routine or dietary insufficiencies. Sometimes, dietary supplements rectify metabolic disorders. For instance, thiamine (B-1) supplementation is utilized under close restorative supervision in the treatment of a few hereditary metabolic disorders, including sub-intense necrotizing encephalopathy, Maple syrup pee infection and hyperalaninemia.

Diabetes is viewed as one of the metabolic disorders in light of the fact that either an absence of insulin or lessened affectability to insulin keeps glucose from entering the phones and being changed over to vitality. Both types I and type II diabetes are in any event in part hereditary.

Researchers trust that they have recognized the quality that inclines a man for type II diabetes, however, notwithstanding when the condition is normal among relatives, legitimate eating regimen, weight loss, and expanded physical action can keep the condition. There is additionally confirm that organic and natural supplements, and in addition, the dietary minerals calcium and chromium might be useful.

In type II, shameful eating regimen and physical idleness prompting focal heftiness is a noteworthy hazard factor. Around 65% of all people with type II diabetes are overweight or large. At one time, type II was alluded to as grown-up beginning diabetes, yet as of now, on account of an expansion in youth heftiness, there has been an increment in type II diabetes among kids.

In most metabolic disorders, there are missing or dishonorably developed proteins fundamental for the generation of vitality in the cell. Hence, at times, compound supplements amend metabolic disorders. In the event that left untreated, metabolic disorders can prompt neuropathies (nerve harm). The nerve harm is caused either by the cells fail to appropriately utilize vitality or by a development of substances inside the body that harms the nerves.

On account of diabetes, uncontrolled abnormal amounts of glucose in the circulatory system make harm the nerves and organs of the body. While glucose isn't regularly lethal and is important for appropriate mind work and unnecessarily low levels can prompt trance state, constantly abnormal states, in the end, wind up poisonous.

Diabetes is a standout amongst the most widely recognized reasons for metabolic neuropathies. Different causes incorporate thyroid illness, hypoglycemia (low glucose) and nutritious insufficiencies. Despite the fact that, nutritious insufficiencies are perceived as the reason for some non-hereditary metabolic disorders. The connection between type II diabetes and sustenance is questionable. Despite the fact that, dietary supplements revise metabolic disorders, there is no settled upon supplement regimen for diabetics.

Numerous specialists and advocates of option and corresponding prescription trust that an entire nourishing supplementation program ought to be intended for diabetes and those in danger for type II diabetes. This is a subject of individual intrigue, on the grounds that a considerable lot of my nieces and nephews are in danger. Originating from a vast family I have seen the infection desolate loved ones, as difficulties created causing the loss of sight, coronary illness and nerve brokenness.

By and by, I am sick of sitting tight for the standard therapeutic group to concur that there are compelling natural and wholesome supplements to battle and keep the entanglements of diabetes. It is likely the most well-known of the metabolic disorders and is perceived as a standout amongst the most widely recognized reasons for metabolic neuropathies, but since insulin infusions can control the sickness to a specific degree, subsidizing for research of option and corresponding pharmaceutical is inadequate.

Lose Weight While Sleeping - Simple and Easy

Get thinner while sleeping isn't something unthinkable. I know it does sound strange to you, how might somebody get in shape while sleeping? For your data, you can accomplish your optimal weight less demanding when you rest soundly and in addition following a specific feast plan.

Essentially, you can get more fit while sleeping because of your hormones. Specialists trust that your hormones are taking part in exercises like consuming fat amid your rest time. This will just happen when you take a particular eating routine amid the day and get great rest during the evening.

You can attempt the menu beneath to assist you with losing weight while sleeping. You should just expend your dinners amid the prescribed circumstances and kindly don't avoid any suppers. Expand more beverages when you are experimenting with this menu however, kindly don't take any sort of bites.

Right off the bat, you should take your breakfast at a young hour toward the beginning of the day, around 6.00 am to 8.00 am. Take some bread with nectar or stick, which one you favored. For drinks, you can take tea, juice or espresso. Breakfast is something which will build your insulin level, yet rest guaranteed that you will remain vivacious for the entire day in the wake of devouring breakfast. Distribute around 5 hours time as a break after your breakfast before you take your lunch once more.

Lunch is presumably the most charming supper for you since you are permitted to eat as much as you can imagine. Be that as it may, endeavor to incorporate more proteins in your sustenance and additionally guides. There are a few choices which you can look over, for example, eating meat with potatoes or pasta with green veggies. You can likewise take dessert for your lunch to fulfill your sweet tooth! Offer yourself a 5 hours reprieve before you go for your supper. It is alright for you to take drinks like water, espresso and tea which have not been sweetened by sugar, drain or different types of sweetener.

Guides are unquestionably out of the rundown with regards to supper on the off chance that you need to get thinner while sleeping. Consequently, you should take out sustenance like pasta, bread, and potatoes from your rundown when you are setting up your supper. Take more proteins by eating fish and eggs and also stack yourself up with vegetables. Plates of mixed greens will be an awesome decision for your supper! This is to keep the body from creating insulin so it can gather during the time spent consuming fat.

Investigate our accumulation of formulas which have been made in view of you. They arrive in an assortment of decisions and top notch and holding your wellbeing and weight in line! This is certainly not some handy solution eat less which you have tired about; this is one online eating regimen program which will assist you in attaining your weight loss objective steadily and normally. Ever Loss can control you well to influence your weight loss to travel a success! Lose your weight reliably and ward off them from your body for eternity.

14 Foods That Speed Up Your Metabolism

On the off chance that you are searching for a rundown of foods that will assist you with speeding up your digestion and influence you to consume more fat, you have gone to the perfect place. While the foods underneath are on the whole sound in their own right, it is insightful not to skirt any nutrition types with the goal that you have a very much adjusted eating design. So let us investigate 14 foods that will get you off to a sound begin on your weight loss design.

1. Apple Cider Vinegar

This is a phenomenal diuretic that you can utilize it as serving of mixed greens dressing. Apples being one of the fixings contains malic corrosive which has fat consuming properties. The aging procedure makes this vinegar need to have helpful acids which consolidate with antacid components and minerals in your body. What this does is create a cell scouring impact. It likewise has elevated amounts of potassium which contains a disinfectant quality, which will kill your fat stores.

2. Asparagus

A concoction called asparagine contained in asparagus is an alkaloid that animates your kidneys, bringing about a superior circulatory process. Alkaloids specifically advances the separating of fat by your phones. It likewise expels squander from your body by separating oxalic corrosive, this corrosive tends to attach to fat cells. By separating this corrosive, it will lessen your fat levels.

3. Beets

Beets have impacts concentrated on your liver and kidneys. Being a solid diuretic beets flush out your skimming body fats. They contain a type of iron that washes down the corpuscles. Corpuscles are platelets with fat stores. There is additionally a little chlorine content that flushes out greasy stores, likewise it likewise invigorates the lymph which gets out the fat stores.

4. Brussel Sprouts

Brussel grows empowers your organs, particularly your pancreas. Your pancreas will then discharge more hormones that cleansingly affects your cells. They likewise contain minerals that fortify your kidneys with the goal that waste is discharged quicker which thusly gets out your cells.

5. Cabbage

The sulfur and iodine in cabbage will wash down your assortment of waste issue, particularly the mucous layer of your stomach and digestion tracts. Cabbage is awesome on the off chance that you need to lose your stomach fat, it will separate the fat here.

6. Carrots

Carotene in carrots is a type of Vitamin A, which begins a fat flushing response in your body. This response accelerates the procedure which your body washes out fat and waste. The change of carotene into vitamin An in your digestion tracts will make a lift in your digestion notwithstanding causing a response whereby your cells expel fat stores.

7. Celery

The high grouping of calcium in crude celery is in a shape prepared for use by your body. As a result of this the calcium will be sent specifically to work. This unadulterated type of calcium touches off your endocrine framework which separates the amassed fat develop. Celery additionally has a high magnesium and iron substance which will enable wipe to out your framework.

8. Cucumber

The high substance of sulfur and silicon in cucumber attempts to empower your kidneys in washing out uric corrosive, which is a waste item. With the evacuation of uric corrosive, fat expulsion is empowered by the extricating of the fat from cells.

9. Garlic

Garlic notwithstanding being a characteristic diuretic likewise contains mustard oils. These oils advances a purifying activity in your body, which empower incredible peristalsis (strong withdrawal), this thus release fat and help to wash out those fats. They additionally help in the breakdown of clusters of fat.

10. Horseradish

Horseradish which is exceptionally mainstream in Japanese dishes has awesome fat dissolving properties and is likewise an incredible purifying operator for your body.

11. Lettuce

The iron and magnesium in lettuce which enters your spleen enable your body to support its resistance and shields yours from getting sick. Your spleen reinforces these minerals and sends them to your cells and tissues. This will help your liver, increment your digestion, and in addition wash out greasy cells. The darker the lettuces, the more the mineral substance.

12. Onions

Having comparable properties with garlic, onions have minerals and oils that assistance to break down fat stores and accelerate digestion also. Onions are more effective and have a milder scent than garlic, it bodes well to add onions to your every day abstain from food.

13. Radishes

The high substance of iron and magnesium in radishes cleans the mucous film of your body, and in addition, help to break up fat in your cells.

14. Tomatoes

Tomatoes are high in vitamin C and additionally citricmalic-oxalic acids. Notwithstanding quickening the metabolic procedure, it additionally causes your kidneys to discharge more water to help wash away fats. The regular acids with the chemical enacted minerals provoke the kidneys to sift through huge amounts of greasy stores which is then dispensed with from your framework. So add tomatoes to your every day eat less carbs and have your digestion thank you for it.

Weight Loss Is Actually Based On the Metabolism

The greater part of the dieticians trusts that getting in shape is in reality about dealing with the digestion of our body. Thus, at whatever point there is any say about the digestion, we have to comprehend that it is the signs towards the best possible eating regimen of people. Besides, it has turned into the discussion of the time nowadays. All things considered, we have to comprehend that the subject of digestion is tied in with becoming more acquainted with the basics of our own body.

In such manner, it has been informed that a human body is an incredible living being which is self-worked and functions according to the characteristic systematic standards. Out of such standards, on is about the rule under which our body tries to accomplish homeostasis or a place of impeccable balance.

Along these lines, if our kid has a flawless balance than, we don't should be on edge about accomplishing its ideal body weight nor we have to consider extreme fats or how to lose it. Likewise, we are free from going on a legitimate eating regimen or any sort of pills for getting in shape. In the meantime, we require not need to experience the daily paper for getting the most up to date weight loss plan or need to remain wakeful to get the late night show of shedding pounds on the TV. All things considered, in the event that we have fulfilled that our body has quite recently the privilege metabolic balance and after that, we don't need to consider any over-burden fat to dispose of.

In this way, we can state that accomplishing this sort of metabolic harmony isn't as intense as it appears. In spite of the fact that, we could discover a few people who might expand a similar procedure in such a route as though keeping up the metabolic harmony will take the whole existence of a man. We have to comprehend that metabolic harmony does not have such kind technique or equation which must be taken after unbendingly. In this way, we should simply to know and mindful of some major laws of nature. Along these lines, we have to keep up a similar law to accomplish the metabolic harmony and that is all.

For this situation, we simply need to recall a portion of these basic, yet powerful crucial laws of nature. Initially, we have to keep up a characteristic eating regimen which would be brimming with protein. Also, we should stick to such administration which involves cardiovascular exercise and weight preparing. Thirdly, we have to take a standard sleeping example each time we rest. Last however not the minimum, that is, we have to control the liquor utilization.

William Brandson

Recommended Daily Amount of Protein - How Much Protein Do You Need Daily to Burn Fat Not Muscle?

Suggested day by day measure of protein admission would vary from individual to individual contingent on their activity levels and bulk. Protein utilization is greatly advantageous for building muscles, bones, skin, and hair. Generally, individuals going to exercise centers, sprinters and weightlifters try to supplant sugars with proteins in their eating routine that can turn out to be exceptionally destructive.

An adjusted eating regimen is constantly fitting for keeping up a great wellbeing. Proteins, as a rule, shield our body from unsafe substances by creating antibodies. It produces helpful compounds and gives bunches of vitality. Eggs lean meats, organic products, green-hued vegetables and soy-based items are the best wellspring of proteins. A great many people likewise take protein supplements for consuming fat. It is constantly prudent to expend 0.83 grams of protein for every one pound of your body weight. Your general eating routine ought to contain 15 percent proteins as per RDA.

Take after these means for estimating your protein needs:

• Step 1: Firstly you should gauge your weight in a measuring machine.

• Step 2: You should isolate your general weight by 2.2 with a specific end goal to change over it in Kgs.

• Step 3: You ought to duplicate your weight (Kg) with 0.8 gm/kg.

• Step 4: This gives you a thought regarding the genuine measure of proteins required by your body.

By following these means, you can undoubtedly choose your prerequisites. It is constantly advantageous to keep up the levels of each supplement in your eating regimen for better outcomes.

Prescribed day by day measure of protein is likewise gainful for development. It is the most favored supplement for youngsters between 8-18 years. Proteins fabricate your muscles as well as help your body in picking up tallness and quality. It takes care of your general wellbeing. You ought to likewise drink heaps of water for accomplishing the most extreme advantages from proteins. You should drink no less than 10-12 glasses of water day by day.

Recommended Foods to Lose Extra Weight

Foods are the wellspring of vitality which the body needs keeping in mind the end goal to work. In any case, indulging may result in elevated amounts of putting away vitality and fats that for the most part prompt overweight and heftiness.

To discharge the putaway vitality, a normal exercise is vital for weight loss and building bulk which advances a speedier metabolic rate. Be that as it may, a dynamic way of life ought to dependably be supplemented with a solid eating regimen to influence the weight loss to program more compelling.

These are probably the most prescribed foods to lose the additional weight:

Fish

Certain fish, for example, fish, salmon, and sardines contain a hormone called Leptin which consumes the putaway vitality and fats coming about to weight loss. Besides this advantage, an angle is high in protein that can settle the glucose and check hunger which at that point forestalls indulging.

Safe starch

Safe starch can be found in bananas, naval force beans, lentils, wholegrain bread, cereal, and potatoes and has been found to expand the muscle versus fat's consuming capacity by 20 to 30 percent.

Like other dietary fiber, safe starch keeps the body from putting away a lot of fats and influences the body to feel full for a more extended period contrasted with different types of sugars.

Flavors

Flavors, for example, cayenne peppers, garlic, hot mustard, hot peppers, and cinnamon can build the muscle to fat ratio's consuming capacity by to 20 percent notwithstanding for three hours subsequent to eating hot foods.

Most flavors likewise contain synthetic compounds which advance the arrival of norepinephrine and epinephrine hormones which at that point lessen the hunger and nourishment desires.

Crude nuts

Nuts have elevated amounts of fiber which can diminish the sentiment of hunger and elevate quicker digestion because of their high measure of Omega-3 fats and protein. In a perfect world, individuals ought to eat crude nuts rather than salted and simmered ones to get the full advantage of such foods.

Crude vegetables and natural products

Crude vegetables and natural products are by and large low in calories than the body consumes more vitality while processing these foods. As per specialists, this negative calorie impact can result in weight loss.

Beside this, crude vegetables and organic products are high in vitamins and minerals which can flush out the body's poison. These likewise contain large amounts of filaments which check the sentiment of hunger.

Dairy products

Yogurt and drain contain a specific substance which changes over the putaway fats into vitality. In any case, to additionally profit from these dairy products, individuals ought to pick the low-fat adaptation.

Choose the Diet Program That Matches Your Personality

The fight with the abundance poundage is a long and dreary process. The attack of various eating regimen programs is doing hurt more than great on individuals who have been attempting to lose weight for whatever length of time that they can recollect. The assortment of alternatives is something worth being thankful for, however, there are times when they can be exceptionally overpowering. This is on the grounds that individuals tend to attempt what is new. You might take after an eating regimen design religiously, yet the energy of promoting can without much of a stretch influence you to lose concentration, particularly on the off chance that you trust that one eating regimen program is by all accounts working more than the other. The essential thing to recollect is that eating routine projects were composed particularly for various purposes.

All things considered, it's likely best to first figure out what your concern is. The answer to your weight issue won't come instantly. You have to assess your way of life and decide the variables that may have added to your weight issue. You don't have to attempt all the diet programs that are being promoted on TV. Much of the time, impact weight misfortune is joined by an eating regimen arrange for that is tailor-fit for your own needs.

It's not possible for anyone to promptly say which eat less arrangement works just by taking a gander at you. It takes a cautious examination of you to discover the great and the unfortunate propensities. When you have recorded down the things that may have added to your weight issue, you can begin window looking for the eating routine projects. It's imperative to do your examination before digging into a particular eating routine arrangement. As there are numerous projects to look over, limit your rundown and pick those that you feel will profit you over the long haul. On the off chance that you just have a couple of projects to browse, you won't need to stress over data over-burden. Simply adhere to those that will coordinate your present way of life and dietary patterns.

Each eating regimen program has an alternate way to deal with helping individuals lose the overabundance weight. You likewise need to mull over your present restorative condition in the event that you are truly considering experiencing an eating routine program. Counseling your doctor before beginning a program will enable you to comprehend your body and your needs. Thusly, you don't subject yourself to any wellbeing dangers. While each eating regimen program has a one of a kind strategy, the fundamentals of abstaining from excessive food intake are typically present on each program. A blend of solid sustenance admission, viable calorie control and exercise are typically part of the majority of the eating regimen programs being offered on the web.

This data isn't something you are not effectively mindful of. What most diet programs do is to help give you the correct instruments and inspiration to get past your weight issues. When you pick an eating routine arrangement that matches your way of life and addresses your weight issue, stick to it for the length of the program. It is just in finishing the specific program you can emphatically say that it works or it doesn't. Try not to be compelled into joining an eating routine program that you feel isn't right for you.

CONCLUSION

Metabolism is apparently a standout amongst the most misjudged ideas among the overall population. How regularly do you hear individuals saying things like 'she should have an elevated capacity to burn calories - that is the reason she can eat anything and still be so thin.' Although this isn't altogether wrong, it is vital to comprehend what metabolism is and how it underpins your body and how it functions for you. Metabolism is only the common procedure through which your body changes nourishment into vitality. Nourishment should be separated from your body to have the capacity to utilize it as vitality. Accelerating your metabolism will clearly accelerate the procedure at which your body changes over sustenance and put away fat into vitality and therefore you 'free weight'.

The regular confusion that such a large number of individuals hold is that they are 'conceived' with either a high or a limited capacity to burn calories. Your hereditary makes up represents just 5% of your metabolic rate. Whatever is left of your metabolism is controlled by none other than you.

There are just two factors that can represent your metabolism. Accelerating metabolism needs to concentrate just on these two zones. Albeit certain genetic components can assume a part we will dispose of them for our dialog (it influences just a little level of individuals at any rate.)

Basically, right off the bat metabolic disorder would cause hormonal irregularity of the endocrine framework. Besides, they exasperate insulin levels. Thirdly, they cause mind-set science disturbances. Fourthly, they cause vitality and safe brokenness. Also, ultimately, it makes candida yeast colonization in mucosal films. Straightforward and apply? You can wager your last dollar!

As the last word, here are a few expressions of supportive gestures. On the off chance that you have been perusing precisely this section, you presumably have more information about the metabolic disorder and weight pick up that do numerous specialists. Learning is control. Along these lines learning about nourishment is control over sustenance that reason metabolic disorder.

Printed in Great Britain
by Amazon

57529548R00050